CBD OIL

A simple & effective beginner's guide on using CBD Hemp Oil, the natural remedy to cure illnesses, improve health, mental health, pain relief, & cure anxiety without medications

Warren Ziesmer

Table of Contents

Introduction

Congratulations on purchasing *CBD OIL: A simple & effective beginner's guide on using CBD Hemp Oil, the natural remedy to cure illnesses, improve health, mental health, pain relief, & cure anxiety without medications* and thank you for doing so.

The following chapters will discuss the growing popularity and different uses of CBD oil. You will learn a bit about the misunderstood history surrounding this natural oil and educate yourself when trying to sift through what many would consider a controversial and almost taboo topic. As knowledge about the multiple health benefits that can be found from using CBD oil continues to grow, more and more people will be turning to it when trying to find an alternative to common modern-day medical treatments. The information you will find in this book does not aim to cause a war between holistic remedies and modern medicine but to find out how to balance the two properly. Even so, you may just discover for yourself that by using CBD oil, you may not need to depend upon just doctors and the medical industry anymore.

You will also learn about the different ways that people use in taking their CBD oil. Health does come first but using CBD oil can turn into a fun hobby!

There are plenty of books on this subject on the market, thanks again for choosing this one! Every effort was made to ensure it is full of as much useful information as possible, please enjoy!

Chapter 1: What Exactly is CBD Oil?

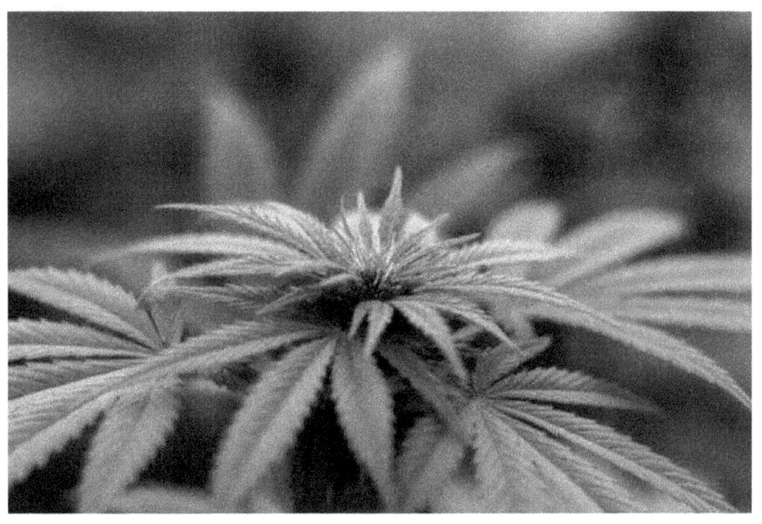

In the year 1940, a new discovery was made. Roger Adams, a graduate from Harvard university who would later in life go on to become a chemist, was successfully able to extract cannabidiol (CBD) from the Cannabis sativa plant. Roger Adams, at the time, was not aware of the importance of the findings he had made. As the years passed by, Roger Adams would eventually come to learn how important his discovery of CBD oil was. He did not work alone or independently in doing so and can't be solely labeled as the only one who helped to bring the benefits of CBD oil to light.

An entire 6 years would have to go by before, in 1946, the first test was conducted using CBD oil on lab animals. This test was conducted by Dr. Walter S. Loewe. Dr. Walter S. Loewe's test revealed that there is no altering of any mental state from the use of CBD oil. Later that same year another test was done, this time it was under the guidance of one Dr. Ralph Mechoulam. Dr. Ralph Mechoulam is often the person that receives the credit for discovering CBD oil. Although he was not the first, Dr. Ralph Mechoulam can take direct credit for learning that CBD's contain a three-dimensional structure which would pave the way for more test and research studies to be done by another scientist. In the 1960's, these other scientists started to catch up with the three trailblazers of Roger Adams, Dr. Walter S. Loewe, and Dr. Ralph Mechoulam, when they started to test CBD oil use on primates. Not too long after the testing of CBD oil in primates, CBD oil was released specifically for therapeutic use by a British pharmaceutical company. Then, in the 1980's, Dr. Ralph Mechoulam ran a paramount study that proved CBD oil could be used as a major factor for treating epilepsy. This was only the start of the long and fascinating history of the health benefits found in using CBD oil. Since then a plethora of ramifications have been confirmed for its medicinal use and as time keeps on ticking, there will surely be more discoveries and therapeutic confirmations to come.

Today CBD oil lingers on the tightrope and razor thin edge that separates controversy from popular acceptance. To receive CBD oil, it must be extracted from hemp or marijuana. This has placed some legal hurdles and obstacles in the way of CBD's use becoming more common, popular, understood, and accepted. All 50 of the United States supplements of CBD oil extracted from hemp are now considered legal. This was not accomplished via a straight and well-lit road though. There have been many detractors, possibly relating to inaccurate propaganda and false understanding related to marijuana and CBD, who were adamantly wanting to keep CBD locked in a cell of demonization and fear. In the year 2014, the United States showed a sweeping cultural breakthrough and change of mindset when several different states gave clearance to passing laws that allowed the use of CBD for medical purposes. These sates were Wisconsin, Utah, Tennessee, South Carolina, North Carolina, Missouri, Mississippi, Kentucky, Iowa, Florida, and Alabama. In other countries, including those that make up the United Kingdom, CBD has also become a legal supplement.

Now that the legal, cultural, scientific, and political worlds have become slightly less adversative to using CBD oil for therapeutic purposes, a variety of different methods and facilities are now in place to harness the healing power of this long misunderstood oil. There are different CBD lotions and waters available, which would have never been the case less than 30 years ago. CBD oil has been promoted to reduce anxiety, remove stress, curb different sorts of aches and pains, lower inflammations, help alleviate depression, and also is said to help minimize or remove the symptoms of maladies, discomfort, and illnesses. There are some groups of people that have even gone so far as to no longer depend upon traditional painkillers, instead opting to fill their medicine cabinets with vials and jars of CBD oil. For people who suffer from mental issues, CBD oil has been shown to help calm down a variety of associated symptoms. Even athletes regularly extol the value of CBD oil, normally rubbing the lotion onto areas of their bodies after a hardy session of exercise. For CBD oil has been around for so long and having its multiple uses and benefits proven several times, it is quite amazing that the oil has to keep providing evidence on how legitimate it really is. In at least some locations, society has softened some of its stance regarding hemp and marijuana, CBD oil has finally been given an easier passage to do some of the things that its best at.

The reason that this has all been happening is because of the cannabinoids that are the molecules found inside the Cannabis sativa plant. These cannabinoids are what gives off the recreational and medical properties related to cannabis. There are over 60 different and unique cannabinoids found in cannabis and CDB is only one of them. The most famous of these cannabinoids is probably tetrahydrocannabinol, most often referred to simply as THC. THC is the substance that brings on the altered state of consciousness (commonly known as "being high") after smoking, or any other method, of ingesting marijuana. Any compound that alters the state of consciousness is known as a psychoactive or psychotropic compound. CBD is a non-psychoactive or non-psychotropic compound, and thus, will not alter someone's state of consciousness. You won't get high from using just CBD oil. Many, if not most, of the different strains of marijuana, have far more amounts of THC then CBD, extracting the CBD oil for therapeutic use has been a difficult task to surmount in the past. As CBD is becoming more accepted, extracting just the CBD without the THC is becoming more common, and will most likely continue in the future.

Legalizing marijuana has become a hot button sort of topic, with people on both sides more than ready to offer up strings of opinions and theories supporting it, even if no one asked them to. Using CBD oil for therapeutic use, however, has almost been, more or less, separated from the debate of legalizing marijuana. You most likely live in an area where using CBD oil is completely legal and safe from legal persecution. If you are, then you are free to experiment with it and see if it can help to alleviate whatever medical condition, may it be physical or mental, that may be ailing you. Finding CBD oil should not be a hard task to complete either, as it is growing in popularity and winding up on more and more store shelves. If you do have trouble locating a store that carries it, then just go look online as numerous websites sell and deliver it. However, if you happen to live in an area where using CBD oil is still frowned upon, then it has to be clearly stated that you should not place yourself in a legally pernicious situation. If that is the unfortunate and unfair circumstances of the area where you live, then you should look for a different holistic and natural alternative to modern medicine aside from using CBD oil. There are also many different types of brands that sell CBD oil, and as such, you should take the time after reading this book to do your own research and learn a little bit more about each brand available.

Also, be aware that the information in this book is not a replacement for your normal health care provider. Doublecheck with your doctor before performing any self-medication, even if it is something as safe and trusted as using CBD oil.

How Does CBD Oil Work?

A common misconception about herbs and plants (or in this book's case a specific compound found within them, specifically CBD oil) is that when they are introduced into the human body, some sort of gross or mystical transmutation takes place and either makes people sick, healthier, or high. The human brain does not exactly work like that. Although much of how the brain works is still not fully understood it continues to be glacially demystified a little bit more each passing year. The questions of yesterday become the answers of tomorrow.

There are substances that are created inside the human body that are called endocannabinoids. Inside the human brain there are a variety of different receptors that allow us to take in stimulus from the external world and not just allow anything to enter our bodies, but actually put to use whatever the external stimulus may be. Think of the antenna attached to your car and compare it to your brain and body. Then think of a radio station located somewhere in the area where you live. That radio station (external world) sends out a stimulus (a song on the radio) and it is received by your brain and its different receptors (the car antenna). Without having receptors in our bodies and brains, all the stimulus from the external world would just pass us by. Without these receptors we would not be able to smell, taste, hear, feel, or even see anything ever.

Endocannabinoids are the receptors in our bodies and brains that are specifically wired into us so that we can receive and notice all the different cannabinoids, such as THC or CBD, that can enter our physiological system. The very first cannabinoid receptor was not discovered until 1998. After it was found to exist within the human body, the scientist went straight to work trying to locate a ligand for the receptor.

A ligand can be thought of as something that binds to a receptor in the human body. After a ligand binds itself to whatever receptor it may be, it can change the way those receptors operate and behave. When THC binds onto a receptor, it will often change the behavior and structure of what it has bonded onto, and since THC is psychoactive, it will bring about the altered state of consciousness. In other words, THC binds and acts as a ligand, binds itself to a receptor in the brain, and alters the receptor so it feels "high".

Then there is CBD. Since CBD is not psychoactive, it will also bind to a receptor but when doing so, there will be no sensation of being high.

When it comes to endocannabinoid receptors, there are two things that are needed to be clarified. CB1 is the first and it is distributed all throughout different regions of the brain. The parts of the brain that they seem to be the most affluent in are the motor functions of the endocrine system (automatic and manual control), cognition, memory, emotion, sensory perception, pain reception, coordination, and anything that includes movement.

The second endocannabinoid receptor to take note of is called CB2. These receptors are mostly located in the immune system. So far science has determined that these receptors mostly affect the reduction of certain types of aches and pains, as well as acting as an anti-inflammatory.

Research continues to prove that CBD does not have a strong effect on either CB1 or CB2 receptors. THC does have a strong effect on both CB1 and CB2 receptors and is also psychoactive. This is a major reason why the majority or marijuana that has been grown for recreational use has a vastly higher amount of THC instead of CBD. So, when using CBD oil, you will receive the health benefits that are found within the extract but will not be activating the parts of your brain that bring on the altered state of consciousness.

When extracting the CBD from cannabis, it will turn into a yellowish looking oil. After it has been turned into a liquid, it can then be added to water or be used similarly to all the other different ways that people use oils.

CBD Oil VS Hemp Oil

There are numerous different oils that can be extracted from the *Cannabis sativa* plant. Marijuana oil, THC oil, cannabis oil, and CBD oil all come from the same source but depending on how the plant is grown, and how the oils are extracted, will determine what types of oil you get and what it can be used for.

When most people refer to CBD oil, they may also call it Hemp oil. This is not an entirely inaccurate name to give it, scientifically speaking. They should not be grouped together though. When referring to hemp oil, it should be called hemp seed oil as that is more specific to what people usually are referring to.

Hemp seed oil has a clear appearance, unlike CBD oil. Without knowing it, you may have used hemp seed oil numerous times before. It is a common ingredient in many different beauty products, and even in some food. Hemp seed oil is known to have all of its own share of assorted benefits and uses. It needs to be made very, unquestionably, clear that hemp seed oil and CBD oil are not the same things even if they are both extracted from the same plant. There are zero amounts of CBD inside of hemp seed oil. To get hemp seed oil, only the seeds are pressed to extract a liquid substance. CBD comes from the plant and not the seeds that will eventually sprout the plant if grown correctly. There are trace amounts of CBD that can be found within the seeds but nowhere near enough to cultivate any particular, practical, or beneficial use from them. Hemp seed oil should not be used or promoted, for having any therapeutic or medicinal uses. However, hemp seed oil gets to shine is in the world of nutrition- that is possibly the only area where it beats out CBD oil. When extracting a compound from the Cannabis sativa plant for the sake of medicine and therapy, CBD oil trumps hemp seed oil in spades.

CBD oil is not just made from any strain of hemp. It comes from a strain that is bred for specific purposes, such as making topicals, nutritional benefits, and increasing fiber. These specific strains of hemp are much lower in THC and much higher in CBD than just any normal hemp plant. Also, when the CBD is extracted into an oil, it is done so from the use of either the entire plant or just aerial parts. The aerial parts are the different areas of the plant that is constantly and completely exposed to and receiving air and oxygen.

A common method for extracting the CBD oil from the cannabis plant is to soak the plant in a carrier oil (typically olive oil) first before doing anything else. This is done to separate the different components of the plant and extract exactly the type of oil you are looking for, in this case being CBD.

Without the THC, there will not be any mind-altering effects that come from any oil extracted from cannabis. Neither hemp seed oil or CBD oil have THC, and if they do, then the amounts would be so low that they would have no effect on even a child and more so on a full-grown adult.

When looking into all the different holistic remedies that are available when trying to move away from the big named pharmacy companies, CBD oil is one of the most heavily talked about substances that can be found. It is still good to know what you are using though and not to confuse one thing for another. It is worth repeating, hemp seed oil and CBD oil are two different compounds that come from the same source and both have their separate uses. If you are new to the world of CBD oil, then not mixing up one thing for another will be crucial in making sure that your knowledge increases at the proper rate and flow.

Why Use CBD Oil, to Begin with?

The world of modern day medicine can be a scary realm to step into. Side effects are abundant. Waiting in an office for minutes, and sometimes hours, on end can ruin all the planning of not just a single day but can throw a monkey wrench into someone's entire week. Doctors, although valuable and are to be respected, can sometimes misdiagnose or start prescribing pills and medicines for situations that may only require a light touch instead of the heavy hand of medication. Insurance companies are quick to increase rates and surprise the unknowing masses with far too many changes in medical plans and ideologies. Going to the doctor can cost more money than some people can afford, and it is not entirely unheard of for someone to go into debt just by visiting a doctor's office a few times, or maybe even just once. In some cases, people would rather skip medical treatment all together and just live with pain and confusion because going to the doctor or finding a way to pay the bills just comes across as illogical and impossible.

Thankfully there are alternatives out there and using CBD oil is just one of many. In the following chapters, we will delve further into how exactly and what CBD oil can be used for. Now that you have become familiar with what CBD oil is, and what it is not, and now that you know a little bit more about why it works the way it does, you should be able to partake in the many health benefits that it has to offer.

Despite the previous warnings and generally hidden downside of going to the doctor, it has to be stated again that this book is not a replacement for your health care provider. Any medical decision you partake in should be decided after speaking honestly with your doctor.

Go ahead and ask them all the questions regarding CBD oil that you want. They should also have some knowledge to share on the subject. When asking your doctor questions about CBD oil, they may try to steer you away from the issue and any thought of you using it all together. Or, they may not. Doctors are just the same as everyone else. They have their flaws as well as their virtues. If a doctor does not know much about CBD oil (or any other topic), then you have to understand that they may feel as if they have walked into a difficult situation.

Imagine that you are a classroom teacher and have a student that asks a question about a topic you know nothing about, but you are supposed to be an authority on. Common human traits will take over and even a doctor may become embarrassed. Then they will either shoot down the idea entirely, telling you that you are just plain wrong for mentioning something like CBD oil, or they may even do something far worse like starting and making up stories and exaggerating what truths they know as they tell you not to ever partake in CBD oil, all the while they keep handing you prescriptions for various medicines. Of course, not all doctors, and hopefully not even most, would do that but they are all just human beings. Some may act this way, or you may catch them on a bad day.

Or the exact reverse may happen. Your doctor may have more knowledge about CBD oil then anyone you have ever met before, but they were not planning on bringing it up to you due to the controversy surrounding its use. Either way, you are the one who may have to break the ice on the topic and get the conversation started. Please don't hold back and be afraid of bringing up CBD oil to your doctor, and even if they don't support it, you should still do your own research.

Remember to take your health seriously in every manner that you can. In the end, it is only up to you who really gets to make the final decision about your body, mind, and health in every conceivable way.

Chapter 2: Types of CBD Oil

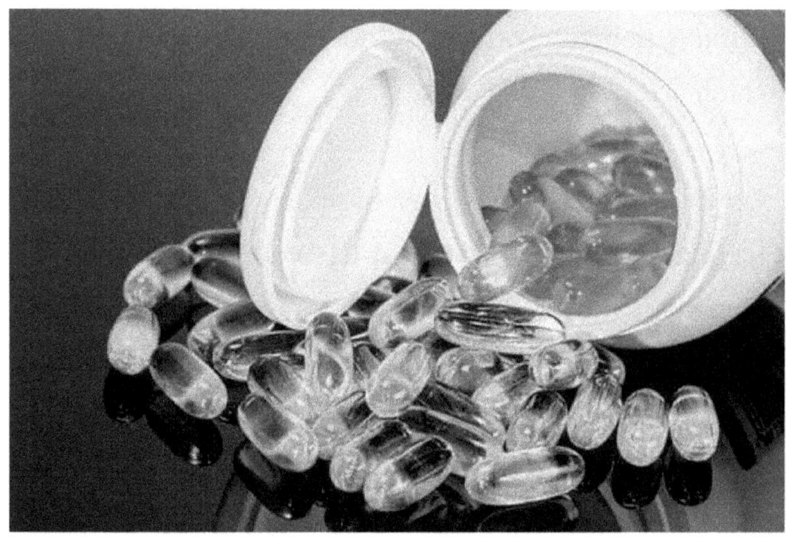

The health benefits from utilizing CBD oil are many and varied. Unlike normal medication where there are exact, at times confusing and impractical, directions for administering them, oils for medicinal purposes usually come much easier, and can even be fun to use. Normally CBD oil extract is taken in the form of a gel tablet or sometimes a pill.

There are other methods and ways to use CBD oil though, and we will go through them for you to help make your understanding and use of the oil even easier. As it was mentioned earlier, using CBD oil will not intoxicate you in any way, although it may make you feel nice, comfortable, sleepy, and bring on a sense of relaxation.

The name of the process for using CBD oil is often referred to as cannabidiol delivery. There are typically four different ways to issue this cannabidiol delivery, and each one of them is safe and easy to understand, while one of them is particularly tasty. Still, each method should be explained to you thoroughly, so you understand what you are getting into.

Don't worry, as you keep on reading I'm sure that you will agree that there is nothing to worry about because the side effects from CBD oil are practically nonexistent, but the more things you know the more empowered you become. Knowledge is power, so they say, and when moving away from the common modern-day medical practices into something more holistic, empowering yourself is really what this is all about.

The Different Methods of Using CBD Oil Medicinally and Therapeutically

Please remember to take note of what type of medical concern you have before using any of these methods. For certain conditions, one way of using CBD oil may be better than another. Also, whatever condition you are dealing with, go ahead and try out a few different methods to see which one works best for you.

And, just in case there are any children or teenagers out there who somehow got this book in their hands, be sure to doublecheck with your parents before using CBD oil or any other herbal substance for medical use or any other reason.

Inhalation

The first method of cannabidiol delivery to cover is inhaling the oil. This should only be done by adults who have a prior history with vaping products like vape pens to replace or replicate cigarettes, standard vaporizers (the type people use to inhale citrus vapors or other fruits) or anything else of the sort. If you are already someone who vapes, then this is a very easy and enjoyable method to get the CBD oil into your system. If you do not have any experience vaping, then you may want to look into some of the other methods listed below. For non-smokers, the process of learning how to inhale correctly will probably come across more as a bother than anything else. Skip the extra complication and move onto the other options. For the sake of clarity, inhaling CBD (or just about anything else next to fumes) usually means that you are smoking it. Again, not to get your hopes up or crush any other ideas you may have- CBD oil does not contain THC and will not get you high- even if you smoke it.

Inhaling CBD oil may very well be the most potent and direct way to reap its benefits. When inhaling it, you will receive more of the original and pure CBD oil than with other methods. When inhaling a cannabidiol it will not just enter the lungs, but the bloodstream. For many of the therapeutic uses for CBD oil, the bloodstream is where you want the oil to go. Any cannabidiol product that enters the human body through this method will very quickly diffuse into the blood and completely bypass the liver and any hemp product that is inhaled will (next to marijuana and TCH) usually exit the bloodstream in only a handful of hours. Although, different results may happen for different people.

There are a vast number of different CBD oils out there that are available for purchase. Going through every one of them would be a herculean task to take on so you will have to try out different ones and find out which type you enjoy. There is a flavor for every sort of person. If you are someone that already has experience vaping, then you should definitely start with this method to begin your journey into the ocean that is CBD oil. If inhaling CBD oil is the way you decide to go, then not only will you be getting all the health benefits, but you may also acquire a brand-new hobby, or just an extension of an old one if you already vape.

For all the parents out there, there is something I want you to keep in mind. Inhaling the CBD oil through a vape is very much akin to smoking, and letting your children get their CBD oil through vaping may teach some habits that you don't want them to start doing later with other things besides CBD. If you are a parent and inhaling CBD is how you decide to get it in your system, it has to be recommended not to have your kids use it the same way, and you may not want to vape in front of them. Of course, this is all preference, and no one has any right to tell someone how to raise their own children, but it still needed to be stated anyway.

Sublingual

The word sublingual means "under the tongue". This method is to be used for CBD extracts that come in the forms of concentrates and tinctures. These mostly only refer to pure CBD oil, so the results will be very fast acting. When placing the CBD oil under the tongue, the capillaries in the mucous membranes will absorb it and send it out into the bloodstream. Then, whatever is left of what you originally placed under your tongue can be safely swallowed. It is also safe to digest and there should be no discomfort. People that have used this method for getting CBD oil into their systems often state that the effects are quick, even immediate, and the results last for a very long time.

The directions for using the sublingual method are beyond easy. For all the parents out there, this may be a good method to get the CBD oil into your child without a whole slew of complaints and headaches. All you need to do is place the CBD under the tongue and keep it there for a minute and a half up to two minutes. After two minutes have passed, the CBD should have been absorbed by the mucous membranes. When going this route, both the digestive system and liver will be bypassed, and the CBD will go straight into the blood, although the tincture that contained the CBT will not, that part will be swallowed and digested. When the CBD oil enters via this method it will find its way to the endocannabinoid system very quickly.

Topical Application

This is a popular one that also serves to soften the skin and start to receive a relaxing sensation even before the CBD begins to take effect. Not only do some CBD topical applications bring a sort of mild and soothing feeling, there are several available on the market that are even used as beauty and skincare products. As CBD oil has risen in popularity even more benefits have been found for it and the transition from CBD topical oil being used for health benefits into the realm of beauty and skincare was almost a no-brainer.

Another great thing about using CBD oil in this way is that it goes straight to work on the concerned part of the body. That's because when using CBD oil topically, it will usually be in the form of a lotion or cream. This makes topical application a popular and thankful way to lessen the pain from stiffness, arthritis, inflammations, and various forms of discomfort to the hands or anywhere else that is needed. It can also help to ease muscles that have been strained or reduce rashes and other skin irritants. Seeing that there is a connection to the world of beauty and skincare, there is also a large variety of different scents and aromas that you can enjoy along with CBD oil applications.

There are just as many types of CBD oil lotions and creams as there are the number of flavors for vaping. This is just another example of how CBD can be used for more than just what it was originally intended for. The benefits of this magnificent oil certainly do seem endless in potential. There have even been something going around on the internet, a little viral item you may have heard of, called the CBD bath bomb.

Ingesting the Oil in a Tablet, Spray, Water, or While Mixed with Food.

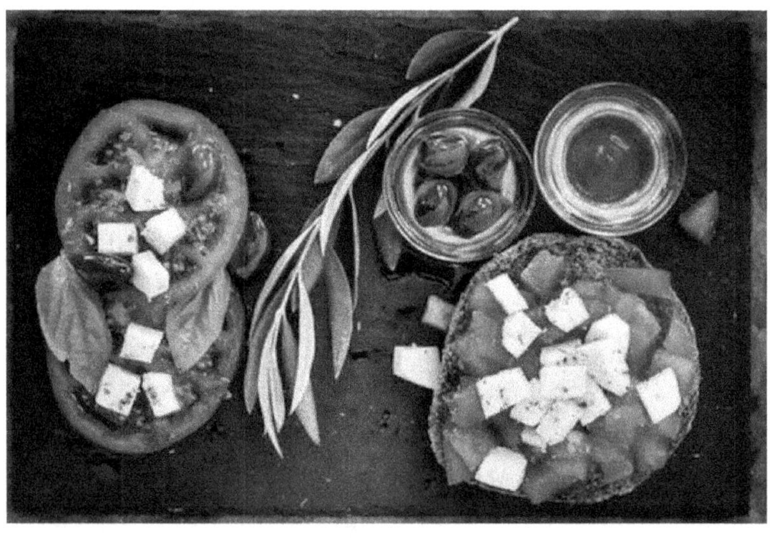

This is the most beginner friendly method for how to get a dose of CBD oil. For those starting out not wanting to use the other methods like children or people that would rather treat their use of the oil quickly like taking a common every day pill, this is the best way to go. Just take a gel like tab or two and pop them in your mouth then swallow it with a glass of water and you're are done with your CBD oil monitoring for the day. Pills concentrate whatever is inside of them which is why they are the standard way of issuing a variety of medicines in the health industry. Even the vitamins we take every day work in this same way and CBD oil pills are no different.

No instruction or training is needed when going this route to get some CBD oil in your system. When taking CBD oil in a pill, it will pass right through the digestive system before entering the liver. Once it has reached the liver it will begin to metabolize. Then the concentrated amount of CBD oil will be released into the bloodstream. CBD oil pills can be treated just as any other supplement out there without worry of side effect or some odd backlash. Just about everyone should be able to swallow the pills without effort or hassle.

Another common method that does not require any training is getting your dose of CBD via a spray. This is not different than any other medical spray. You simply spritz a tiny amount in your mouth and the spray will act similar to a pill. This can be another method used for people who do not have much experience or are a little shy to dive into some of the other methods. Using a spray is also easy to monitor your CBD oil intake.

There are still more ways on how CBD oil can be directly ingested. One of the more simple and common methods is to simply mix the CBD oil with water. These products can be bought at a store or you can mix the oil together with the water yourself. Either way is fine. This method should work well for people who are always on the move and just can't find much time to slow down. If you mix CBD oil into the water on your own, all you have to do is make sure that you have the dosage right and make sure that you drink all of the water throughout your day. That's it! Then you can carry it around with you and drink at your own leisure without bothering to break anything down into a timetable. This is also a popular method of ingestion among athletes, who tend to treat CBD oil the same way they would a bottle of Gatorade or any other electrolyte supplement. If your life is fast paced and you are always zipping from one place to another, then you should begin to use CBD oil via this route.

Taking a pill or spray is not the only way to ingest CBD oil though. It can also be directly mixed with food and consumed by eating. It is completely up to you if you want to go this direction when using CBD oil, but it's something you may want to try at least once. Who knows, maybe you will find a new delicious topping to add to your favorite dishes. Some of the more creative people out there have come up with all sorts of different ways to add CBD oil to food. If you were curious to give this a try, then we have a few ideas that might get your whistle wet.

- Mix CBD oil with pesto and add it to a pizza.
- Add some CBD oil to a fruit smoothie and get a refreshing glass of health! To increase the herbal prestige of the drink, make a smoothie with wheatgrass.
- Combine some CBD oil with chocolate and let your taste buds have a little fun. Truffles go great with CBD oil.

- Beer. Yup, despite knowing that CBD oil doesn't have THC, you can still have a little bit of fun while getting the health benefits of the oil. Hops and cannabis are actually related, so the idea of keeping it in the family of nature isn't too much of a stretch.

- Pour some CBD oil in your coffee to get your morning started.

- Next time you sit down to watch a movie, why don't you switch out the butter for some CBD oil?

- When cooking any number of dishes using olive oil, just simply add some CBD oil to the mix. Many people and chefs have already made this a common practice and its reputation is probably only going to continue to grow.

- There are also different candies and gummies on the market that contain CBD in them.

How Do You Want Your Oil?

As you can see there are plenty of different ways for you to use CBD oil. All these methods serve different purposes and when moving into using CBD oil to help with pain, mental, and physical health issues, using the right type of method will be important. Immediate addition of CBD into your system like the pills and food will work best. Placing CBD oil under the tongue as well will also act in a similar manner to ingesting it. For calming the nerves and placing the brain into a better state of mind, the topical ointments and inhaling it may work better. Using the correct fashion is going to be related to what sort of problem you are trying to reduce. If you have several different problems, then combining some of these methods should help you find a better state of overall health.

Chapter 3: Using CBD Oil Against Illness

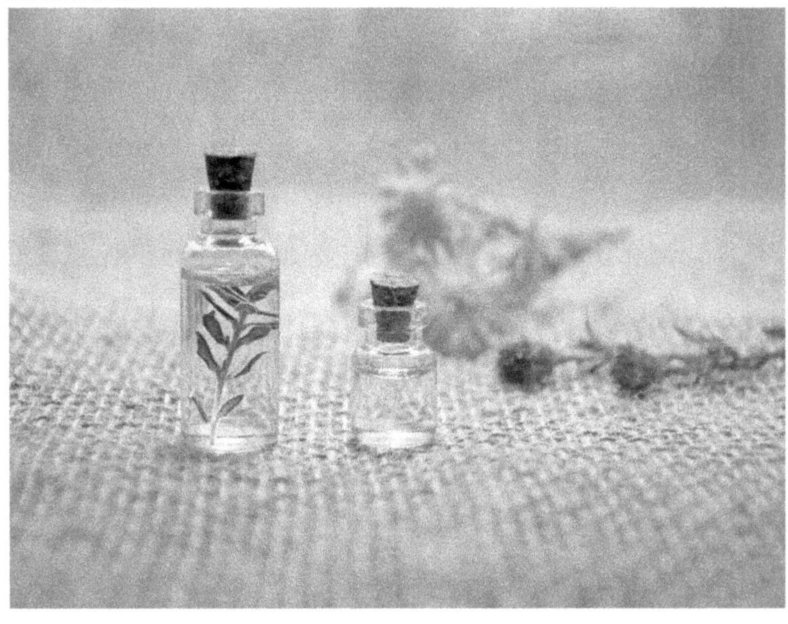

Now that you know a bit more about what CBD is, how it works, and the different ways that you can take it, you can begin to use CBD oil for what it does best. There are several different conflictions and conditions that CBD oil can help to alleviate.

When using CBD oil for the purpose of health it is important to know what sort of result you are looking for. The word "illness" can be broad and at times vague. There are three different types of illness's that any person can be dealing with. They can be physical, mental, and disease. Pain falls under the label of physical illness. Stress, anxiety, and neurological disorders fall under the label of mental illness. For everything else, many of the more common medical conditions that people justifiably fear and don't want to talk about for very long, fall under general illness and overall health.

Being diagnosed with a disease is never easy to deal with. A general illness can take a toll on body, mind, and will often have a domino effect of negativity on not just the person who has unfortunately been diagnosed with a disease, but on the other people around them as well. Using CBD oil is not a magic trick. It is not a mystical herb that will cure all sickness and the rest of life's problems just by using it once or twice. It is to be used in conjunction with the necessary lifestyle changes, instructions provided by a health care provider, and whatever medicine or procedures that may be called for to help combat against the illness in question.

Do not be confused and think that the medical industry is something evil. Wholistic herbs and cures are coming up on the rise and the medical field, being an industry with a whole slew of money wrapped up in it, is simply rebelling against something else moving in to take a piece of the pie. There is no reason to think that common medical practices shouldn't be combined with CBD oil or any other natural treatments.

As more holistic remedies are proven and become accepted, the medical field will be forced to incorporate them into the everyday practices. Many of the bigwigs and suits that determine people's healthcare are not exactly on the side of CBD oil and holistic treatments, but the doctors and nurses that do the real-life field work and provide care for patients have chosen their profession with the best of intentions and should be trusted. Speak to them about using CBD oil. They are the people that are closest to you that know what is going on with your health, and when combining modern medical knowledge with holistic treatments, you will be getting the best of both worlds that can be offered from both sides of the medical spectrum.

The Illnesses that CBD Oil Can Be Used to Fight Against

Since CBD oil, though not new, is still on the rise for medical use there are some areas that have an array of hard data, while others are lacking. Despite this difference in the spectrum, CBD oil has already been shown to help fight against many different sorts of diseases and general health issues. For some diseases, CBD oil can directly fight back against specifically what is wrong, while in other cases it will only reduce symptoms. Both of these, the great and small, aspects and advantages of CBD oil can carry a bit of extra weight when trying to find a way of improving overall health. In the pursuit of becoming healthier, every little bit can add up.

Cancer

One of the first big names that pop up when people begin to use CBD oil is cancer. Although research currently remains in the earlier stages for understanding how CBD can help stave off cancer, results have been promising so far. The National Cancer Institute has leapt into the issue of trying to find out how effective CBD oil is against fighting off cancer. They are not yet willing to completely endorse CBD oil, or anything related to cannabis, for preventing or stopping the growth of cancer cells but they also haven't ignored the positive data that has come in either. It is proven that CBD oil can act as an anti-inflammatory and can also change how certain cells reproduce themselves. Tumor cells are included in this. Early reports have pointed in the direction that CBD oil can reduce the size of some tumor cells as well as stopping them from reproducing altogether.

Breast cancer has been specifically highlighted and has shown to be the most promising regarding CBD oil. A study that was done in 2006 showed, for the first time, that CBD oil could selectively inhibit different growths of breast tumor cancer cells. These were potent effects that could not be disregarded or ignored. When tested on non-cancer cells, the effects were far less potent which lead to the understanding that CBD oil directly fights the cancer cells specifically. CBD oil is thought to possess both pro-apoptotic and anti-proliferative effects which can cause cancer cell migration to inhibit, invasion, and adhesion.

Another research study that was done in 2011 and gave the world a deeper set of data to work with. The researchers learned that CBD oil can induce death directly to tumorous breast cancer cells without harming other tissue. A dependent and concentrated death of the cells located on two important receptors (estrogen receptor-positive and estrogen receptor-negative) was found to take place when CBD oil was introduced to the cells. Since the concentrations of CBD had a very little effect on the mammary cells and other non-tumorigenic ones, this was great news. It more or less showed that using CBD against breast cancer, the other parts of the body that were not showing tumors or symptoms did not suffer side effects. Results of a separate study showed that for people who were suffering from pain related to cancer and not receiving relief from other medication, using CBD oil gave significant relief.

There has also been data gathered that has given support to using CBD oil to overcome not just cancer directly but also help with symptoms related to the disease and the side effects of chemotherapy treatments. Two of the major side effects related to chemotherapy like vomiting and nausea can both be reduced by taking CBD oil.

The current recommended dosage for using CBD to combat against cancer is 700 milligrams taken once a day for 6 weeks straight. No toxicity was noticed with this dosage, leading many to believe that CBD oil can be used as a part of a long-term treatment plan.

Although many of the tests that have been done in relation to CBD oil and cancer have been on lab animals, and more human data is needed before claiming anything as undeniable fact, breast cancer is not the only cancer that may have a weakness to CBD oil. Colon, lung cancer, and leukemia may also be easier to overcome by adding CBD into a treatment plan. As CBD continues to become accepted, the human data that is needed will continue to come in.

Diabetes
It has been proven that CBD can reduce the incidence of diabetes in mice. Up to 56 percent of a reduction of inflammation has been achieved. Also related to

studies involving mice, it has been shown that CBD can reduce plasma levels of proinflammatory cytokines.

Some research has been done on humans as well. One, in particular in 2013, was performed to see what connection, if any, there was between the use of marijuana and insulin, insulin resistance, and glucose. A number of 4,657 different people participated in the test that lasted from 2005-2010. A portion of 1,975 of the participants were former marijuana users and 579 were still using the substance at the time of the study. By the end of the study, it was shown that the people who continued to use marijuana exhibited a 16 percent drop in insulin levels across the board. It was also noticed that the people who were still using marijuana had smaller waistlines. At first, that was not something that much credence was given to but having a larger circumference around the waist can be an onset of diabetes. Like cancer, as time goes by, more human testing and hard data will continue to come to help in connecting the dots between CBD oil and overcoming diabetes.

Heart Health

A direct link has been made between using CBD oil and reducing blood pressure. A small-scale study was done with 10 male volunteers. They were only given a single dose of 600 milligrams of CBD oil. Every one of them had a reduction of blood pressure from using the CBD oil. The researchers running the study then probed a bit farther. The 10 male volunteers were given stress tests that usually leave people having higher rates of blood pressure after they are finished. It turns out that the single dose they took of CBD oil helped them during these stress tests. By the end of the stress tests, the volunteers only showed a slight increase in blood pressure as opposed to the normal rate of increase.

Lowering of blood pressure is a benefit for the entire cardiovascular system, and that includes the heart. If high blood pressure is lowered, so are the risks of metabolic syndrome, heart attack, and having a stroke. Also, there is a less talked about a condition called vascular hyperpermeability (which can cause leaky gut) and that has also been shown to be reduced by CBD oil. CBD oil can also help scrape away whatever excess cholesterol that may have built up in someone's body.

In tests involving animals, CBD oil has shown similar results relating to overall cardiovascular health. Both cell death that is connected to heart disease and inflammations have been known to be reduced in mice that have had CBD oil given to them. It has also been shown to reduce oxidative stress, and even prevent heart damage from spreading wider in mice.

Acne

Although acne may not be as serious an issue as the others in this chapter, it is still a common problem that many people have to struggle with. This is not just exclusive to teenagers either. Many adults have to deal with living with acne on a daily basis. Thankfully CBD oil can help with that as well.

There are several different reasons that can cause acne to rear its ugly head. Bacteria and genetics are two of the more common ones. Yet acne can also be caused by inflammations. As noted, CBD oil is a great anti-inflammatory and it can help to shrink down the cytokines that may be causing acne to develop.

Another major cause of acne is something called sebum. When the body produces more sebum then it needs, there can be a physiological backlash that leads to glands releasing an oily substance throughout the skin. This can be directly counteracted by using CBD oil. CBD can act to lower and slow all sebum growth, thus lessening the appearance of acne.

Other Diseases

The maladies listed in this chapter are the ones where hard data has already been gathered. Even if more hard data is still needed to learn more of the benefits of using CBD oil, the path of knowledge has begun to open up and only more time is needed. Those are not the only medical conflictions that CBD has been shown to help overcome though. There are plenty more.

- CBD oil has been shown to increase appetite.

- Lower inflammations in bowel related diseases such as Crohn's disease and ulcerative colitis.

- Reduce glaucoma.

- Alleviate pain connected to multiple sclerosis.

When used in conjunction with your current treatment plan, CBD oil can help give you that extra kick you may need to help overcome whatever medical difficulty you may be struggling with.

Chapter 4: Using CBD Oil to Curb Pain

Natural pain relief is what has placed CBD oil directly on the map. Among the many advocates who promote the use of CBD oil, alleviating pain is the number one argument and defense they will present. This shouldn't come as some sort of earthshattering surprise. Marijuana, in general, has been used to reduce pain long before any doctor ever prescribed the first medically charged pill. Using marijuana to reduce pain has been recorded as far back as 2900 BC. Although THC probably does play into this to at least some extent, the more prominent reason marijuana is capable of reducing pain can be linked to it being the carrier of CBD oil.

Remember the endocannabinoids that were mentioned earlier? These compounds do more than just regulate what gets bound to the receptors in your nervous system. They also play a part in regulating the response of the immune system, inducing sleep, controlling rate of the appetite, and sensing or dulling pain. When endocannabinoid receptors start firing, pain should lessen. They can sense that there is pain somewhere in the body and go straight to work making the pain less noticeable.

A study that was done on rats helped to prove this point even more. The rats were given slight surgical incisions. They were then given a dose of CBD oil. Low and behold, the rats showed a reduction in the sensation of pain and instead of wallowing in pain, they returned to their normal behavior faster than normal. A separate study that was also done with rats was in relation to inflammation and sciatic nerve pain. These rats were given oral CBD oil treatments. Just like the rats who received the surgical incisions, the rats who received the oral CBD oil dosages returned to normal behavior sooner than they would have otherwise.

As far as studies on humans go, a few of those have been conducted as well. Most of them have been done examining what benefits CBD oil could offer to people who were suffering pain caused by rheumatoid arthritis and multiple sclerosis. Several countries all over the world have already cleared CBD oil for reducing pain for people who have those conditions.

When over 40 different people (who all had multiple sclerosis) were gathered for a research study, they were all given a dosage of CBD oil through an oral spray. This test lasted for an entire month. The results came out as everyone involved had hoped they would. The participants in the study reported that they felt a significant reduction of pain compared to other groups in the study that were given different placebos than CBD oil. The specifically targeted realms of pain that were looked into for this study were muscle spasms and difficulty walking. For all the different people, out there that are unfortunately living with multiple sclerosis, you can take notice that there have been others who reported that using CBD oil has helped them to walk and live a little easier. A few nations out there have already gotten ahead of the CBD medical game by allowing CBD oil to be used in treatment for pain caused by multiple sclerosis. Among these nations, Canada and the United Kingdom are leading the global game and waiting for the rest of the world to catch up with the pack. There are still some debate going back and forth on this issue. It is not yet known if CBD oil acting on its own is the lone agent for alleviating the chronic pain connected to multiple sclerosis. Many of the CBD oil delivery systems that Canada and the United Kingdom use also contain THC.

It may mostly be the CBD oil that helps to reduce chronic pain, but the THC may also be playing a factor in the formula. Either way, CBD oil has been shown to work more than once for removing the chronic pain of multiple sclerosis. There may be a day when the different cultures of the world unite together to get to the bottom of figuring out what all the benefits of the *Cannabis sativa* plant are, instead of breaking everything apart and causing more mysteries and debates, but for now in most countries CBD oil and THC will have to be acquired separately. If the area you live in has an adverse opinion of THC, or if it is just flat out illegal, then you will still be able to gain some comfort from using just straight and pure CBD oil.

The National Institutes of Health have at least dived into learning a little bit more about CBD oil. They took a good look at what could be some of the different ways to alleviate pain from using chemotherapy. It should be clearly identified why chemotherapy is used in the first place. Chemotherapy is used to fight, remove, and kill cancer cells. There is no other reason for someone to use chemotherapy, and as heart breaking that it is to say, chemotherapy can be very taxing for a patient to go through. It does not just attack cancer but can also cause immense pain to the patient during their recovery process. Thankfully CBD oil has shown a bright side to the painful side effect of chemotherapy. It has been reported that people who have undergone chemotherapy have mentioned that they have felt an improvement after using CBD oil. Because of this, adding CBD oil consumption along with chemotherapy is becoming a more common trend.

For people who have been diagnosed with rheumatoid arthritis, similar results have been confirmed. It has been reported that for people who deal with rheumatoid arthritis on a daily basis, they have cited feeling better after taking a dose of CBD oil. Not only has it been shown to reduce the pain and stiffness of arthritis but many people who deal with the affliction have claimed that CBD oil also helps them to sleep better at night. This is not simply isolated to people who can't sleep because of arthritis. Anyone who has difficulty finding a good night of sleep can also use CBD oil for this purpose.

Insomnia is one of the most common medical conditions in the history of humanity. Around a third of the entire population, at any given era in history, are finding trouble sleeping at night due to insomnia. Lack of getting the proper sleep and insomnia may directly cause pain, but every single cell and part of the body acts as an interconnected web. If one area is bothered by something, then there will be a domino effect that will cause a problem somewhere else in the body. Even if a lack of sleep does not directly introduce pain, it sure isn't helping anyone to be healthier than they would be if they did get the proper sleep. Also, when there is a lack of sleep, the human immune system may get confused and not work correctly. Even worse, during sleep, the cells of the human body repair themselves at a much more efficient rate and when not getting the proper sleep, any pain you may be suffering from will only take longer to heal and correct itself. This is another reason to add CBD oil into your cabinet and stop using all the pills that are prescribed far too quickly and in surplus. If you are getting deeper, longer, uninterrupted sleep, you will feel less pain overall, and CBD oil could be just the ticket you need to catch a comfortable ride into dreamland.

In other cases, CBD oil has become something that those who can't waste a single second have come to rely upon. Paramedics, surgeons, doctors, and several different jobs within the medical industry can find themselves in sudden situations that are literally life or death for a patient. Emergencies happen even though we all wish they wouldn't. For people who work in emergency situations, there just is not enough time to think, wonder, estimate, judge, and hope that everything just works itself out. When someone needs emergency medical attention immediately, pain relief must be issued swiftly and effectively. Along with morphine and other ultra-quick acting drugs, CBD oil has been added to the list of emergency medicines that are used for these direst of real world circumstances and situations.

Aside from multiple sclerosis, the side effects of being treated by chemotherapy, rheumatoid arthritis, and emergency pain relief, there are still other areas where CBD oil is currently being looked into for reducing chronic pain. General muscle pain and pain stemming from the spinal cord may be the next wave of darkness where CBD oil can spread some much-needed light. As CBD oil continues to prove itself more and more, the research studies will keep coming and we will surely keep finding new ways to solve some of the oldest and most painful problems.

Aside from some of the more serious and debilitating chronic pains that have been mentioned, CBD oil can also be used for lesser aches and irritations. The topical ointments and applications that were mentioned in chapter 2 come deeply into play here. Just from living a normal life, day in and day out, any single person can start to feel a large variety of different pains. These can happen due to playing sports, stretching wrong, gaining weight, growing old, or sometimes for seemingly no good reason at all. If anything like any of those ever happens to you, then you can rub some CBD oil on the area in question and begin to feel relief almost instantly.

A more infamous example of CBD oil being used to quickly reduce pain and immediately show results have been displayed by an unsuspecting source. MMA fighter Nate Diaz is an avid fan of the substance. Most wouldn't argue that being a pro fighter would lack knowledge on how to handle and regulate pain. I am no MMA fighter, but when one of them talks about how to overcome a variety of pains, you better bet that I'm going to listen. Nate Diaz can regularly be seen vaping CBD oil and has even done so right after a fight has ended, even while the post-match press conference was still going on.

Though some have villainized him for promoting CBD oil so heavily and shamelessly, again, if someone who fights for a living is using it to overcome pain, then it has to work pretty well. Also, no one is going to say that Nate Diaz is out of shape or not in tiptop health.

Of course, his diet, history, genetics, and training regimen all have something to do with this, but CBD oil seems to be working for him quite well. Nate Diaz and his use of CBD oil is just another example of how great the stuff works and what someone could aspire to achieve by adding the oil to their life.

Chapter 5: Using CBD Oil for Mental Health and Anxiety

As harrowing as living with pain and physically debilitating conditions can be, mental pain can be just as challenging if not more to live with. Remember that there is a trifecta when it comes to medical afflictions. There is physical pain, disease, and mental health. For a large number of people out there who have to wake up every single day and muster through a world where their mental health is not working to its maximum ability, CBD oil is there for them as well.

Epilepsy

Epilepsy was the very first medical condition that CBD oil was proven to work well combating against. When someone has epilepsy, they are prone to having seizures and there are areas of their brain that are susceptible to excitability. It just so turns out that cannabinoids, after entering the bloodstream, attach to the specific brain cells that handle the area of excitability that can cause seizures. By doing this, excitability in the brain can be regulated and to an extent controlled enough to reduce seizures from continuing to happen. This is another area where more hard data is needed. When it comes to the medical field, there is never such a thing as having enough hard data, the more information there is at hand, the better it will be for everyone. Yet even the American Epileptic Society has jumped on board in trying to understand how CBD oil can be used to reduce the symptoms and seizures caused from epilepsy.

There was a study done in 2016 which had over 200 people who all were dealing with epilepsy. The participants were given oral dosages of CBD oil every day. The dosages ranged between 2-5 milligrams. For 12 weeks the participants were monitored for any indication of negative side effects, as well as having the rate of their seizures chronicled. For over 70 percent of the participants, their seizures were reduced by almost 40 percent.

Another study was done by Stanford University. This study specifically asked, via the internet, the parents who had children with epilepsy to step forward. The reason they asked this is to acquire volunteers who were willing to see if CBD oil would offer any positive benefit to children with epilepsy. Nineteen different volunteers were found, and the test was sent underway to begin. The average number of drugs that were used to treat epilepsy for the volunteers before volunteering for the test was said to be 12. While it was concluded that being more alert and having an increase in better moods were noticed, what was more satisfying for all involved was the lessening of epileptic problems that were reported. Six of the volunteers said they had a reduction in seizures ranging between 25-60 percent in reduction. Eight volunteers reported an even greater increase in seizure reduction of about 80 percent. Most startling of all, two volunteers reported that their seizures had ceased to happen altogether!

Anxiety and Depression

This is one area where there is practically zero debate. CBD oil works to reduce anxiety and works very well. For anyone who is dealing with social anxiety disorder, CBD oil will help you overcome it. Other sorts of anxiety that are currently being looked into with CBD oil are panic disorder, post-traumatic stress disorder (PTSD), depression, obsessive compulsive disorder, and others.

CBD oil can release dopamine into your system. By doing this, a sensation of happiness will follow. It has also been shown to reduce all sorts of different nervous tension. If you do not have any particular medical ailment, then CBD oil can still be used on a stressful day to take a break from it all and just calm down. Not only can CBD oil release dopamine, but it can also alter the way that the receptors in your brain interact with serotonin. Serotonin is a chemical that is directly connected to all areas of mental health. The bottom line is that when serotonin is moving freely and not inhibited incorrectly, you will let the water of stress roll right off your shoulders.

A study conducted in 2011 focused on public speaking for people who had a social anxiety disorder. Twenty-four people who had the disorder were selected. Some of them were given CBD oil, while others were given other placebos. This was done about an hour and a half before the participants were to attempt public speaking. The results were as predicted. For the people who were not given CBD oil exhibited a higher amount of anxiety, discomfort, and cognitive impairment. For the people who were given CBD oil, they showed more focus and drive while giving their speeches which indicated that the CBD oil helped to calm them down and center them on the task at hand.

A major and longstanding problem that comes along with trying to treat any form of anxiety or depression is the medications that are used to get rid of it. These medicines are all given with good intentions, but the side effects connected to them can actually have the exact opposite effect of what those good intentions are trying to do. First of all, many antidepressants can become addictive and when someone wants to stop taking them, they will quickly see that they just can't stop reaching for the bottle of pills. Then the depression may return, and in the end, the patient has come completed an entire circle and wound up exactly where they began in the first place. Not only can this create a worrisome cycle, but when the pills are removed someone may slip into an even deeper state of depression than the one they started out in, to begin with.

Even though CBD oil can help to overcome the mentally debilitating condition of depression there is no true cure to depression except for one: the patient has to overcome either a traumatic event or something that has altered their personal paradigm and led them into the depressed state, to begin with. This can be one of the greatest challenges that any man or woman can ever face, and many just don't have the strength to see the battle through to the end. For a person to no longer feel depressed, they need to change the way that their brain operates. They need to have more positive chemical production within their brains that can cultivate more positive feelings.

I will not delve in much farther on how such a difficult process is accomplished since that is not the point of this book. However, it should be made very clear that even though CBD oil can help to calm you down and even balance you out, any form of depression that someone may be going through should not be handled solely by the patient. Work with a therapist of some sort. If the price of a therapist is too high and out of your financial reality, then talk to a family member or friend.

If that can't be done, then read a book on the topic, speak to someone online, look into other people's stories and see how they changed their human paradigm into one that is less depressed. Change something about your lifestyle, do something besides just slogging through the uphill battle all alone. CBD oil can help alleviate depression, but to entirely defeat it, you will have to change something else about your life as well. It can be done- please don't ever forget that.

However, since CBD oil has been shown to calm nerves and muscles, tension can be reduced which can start to open up the door to leaving depression behind you. CBD oil can also help you to get better sleep which can go a long way towards helping someone find a better frame of mind.

For anyone who has been diagnosed with PTSD, using CBD oil in conjunction with seeking the help of a mental healthcare professional has shown to reduce anxiety and reduce tensions.

Stroke

Having a stroke can be one of the most frightening things that any single person can ever have to endure. Thankfully, CBD oil has shown to help people that have had the misfortune of having to go through this. CBD can actually reduce the size of the area of the brain that the stroke attacked! By doing this, CBD oil can act as a sort of a shield and continue to protect the brain from getting worse after having a stroke. Similar findings with CBD oil have also been connected to concussions.

Neurological Disorders

CBD oil may also slow down the growth and spreading of Alzheimer's disease. Though many things about Alzheimer's disease remain a mystery, it is known that amyloid plaques are somehow connected to it. Active chemicals in cannabis oil can prevent amyloid plaques from developing.

CBD oil has also shown promise when trying to remove people from substance dependency. Due to a neurological phenomenon called neuroplasticity, CBD oil can help to literally rewire the brain and by doing so, can replace some of the circuitry that has caused someone to remain addicted to a narcotic drug. Tests have only been done on animals thus far, but rats who were tested showed less of a dependency for heroin and morphine after being given a dose of CBD oil.

Also remember that CBD oil is a potent anti-inflammatory, and as such, can help with a number of different neurological disorders.

For people that have been afflicted by Parkinson's disease, CBD oil has shown to help when it comes to getting better sleep. Not only have a few people who live with Parkinson's disease reported that CBD oil can help to reduce pain, they have also claimed that it can reduce night tremors. Others have said that motor skills may also show overall improvement. However, Parkinson's disease is one of the gray areas for CBD oil use. Although CBD oil is not known for having a hefty amount of side effects, and though some people who have Parkinson's disease have said that it has helped them, others who suffer from the disease have claimed the exact opposite. In some small cases, people with Parkinson's disease have actually said that after using CBD oil, their spasms, muscle movements, and night tremors only got worse. More hard data is needed between CBD oil and Parkinson's disease before full confidence for recommending CBD oil can be given.

Antipsychotic

More hard data is needed relating to how effective CBD oil can be when countering issues of mania. Schizophrenia often gets the spotlight here. According to some sources, the pharmacological profile of CBD oil can be classified to be very similar to that of any other atypical antipsychotic drug. As with many of the tests that have been done, most have been on animals, but they still show a hope that CBD oil may one day be the secret key to setting someone with a fractured psyche on the better path to mental health.

This is similar to depression. You should not simply assume that using CBD oil will cure whatever mental disorder you may have. Please seek out the proper professional help if you are dealing with a confused interpretation of reality. It sure can help but discovering the root of your problem and working up from there is the only surefire way to locate all the puzzle pieces of a slightly fractured mind before it can be put back together again. I refuse to extol a false truth and pretend that I understand what living with any form of mania is like and will not insult anyone's intelligence by pretending otherwise. Start by using the CBD oil, but also seek other help if you think that you need it. There should always be a source you can turn to if you truly desire the help enough.

Chapter 6: CBD Oil Roundup

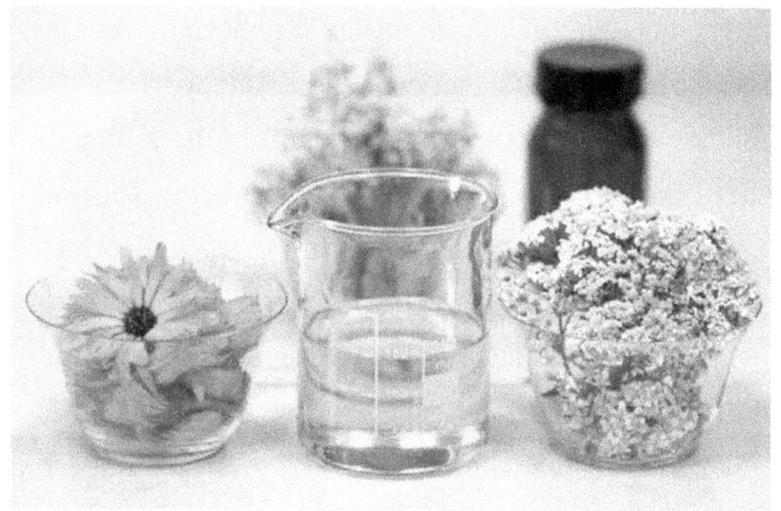

Thank you for making it this far. That is not a trite complaint, but a genuine showing of appreciation. When living with any sort of pain or medical condition, even accomplishing the simplest of tasks like reading a book is no small feat to those that have accomplished them. Go ahead and congratulate yourself, for there is no such thing as a small achievement.

When first stepping into the world of CBD oil, all the options and information can be somewhat intimidating. Hopefully, you have come to see that there is not that much to be worried about. The side effects using CBD oil are minimal and, in many cases, may not even be noticed. You might receive an increase in appetite, and you may become sleepy, but there are far worse things in life then being a little bit hungrier and tired. Other common side effects that have been reported are the sensation of being light headed (though nothing like being high), dry mouth, and a lowering of blood pressure. For many people out there, having the blood pressure lowered should not even be considered a side effect.

There are some side effects that can happen though. Women who are pregnant or currently breastfeeding a baby may not want to use CBD oil. There is no concrete evidence that doing so may be harmful to the upcoming mother or child, but reliable information is lacking for how safe it may be as well. What is known though is that it is common for several different herbs to be harmful to women who are breastfeeding or pregnant.

The one area where CBD oil may not be recommended, and the side effects can actually make things worse is Parkinson's disease. Many who suffer from Parkinson's disease claim that it has helped them to get better sleep, deal with fewer spasms, and have an overall increase in controlling their motor movements better. But on the opposite side of the spectrum, the exact opposite has been stated and some people who have used CBD oil because they have Parkinson's disease have reported that it has actually made their night tremors and muscle movements while trying to sleep worse. Seeing that more hard data is needed on the effects of CBD oil in Parkinson's disease, it may be better to look for an alternative holistic solution to help combat the disease besides using CBD oil.

Dosage amount

CBD oil is not hard to monitor, and some people just habitually use it without paying attention to how much they are intaking. This is common for people who vape with it. For mixing with food and water, follow the directions that come along with a recipe or look on the bottle of water for the recommended dose. Follow the directions for any tablet that may be placed under the tongue or swallowed as well. When using it for a specifically medical reason, 300 milligrams a day is the most common recommended dosage. This amount of CBD oil can be used for up to 6 months without having to deal with any backlash. For higher amounts of CBD oil, about 1,200-1,500 milligrams a day, only use the CBD oil for 4 weeks before taking a break from it. For more delicate issues, consult with your doctor to figure out the right amount of CBD oil that you should be using, and for how long you should continue to use it.

Since you have done so well reading this far, and since we can assume that you want to get straight into using CBD instead of reading the entire book again from the very beginning, a handy and comprehensive list has been compiled for you to use as a quick guide to giving answers to some of the more common CBD oil related questions.

Who were the trailblazers that helped pave the way for CBD oil being used medically?

- Roger Adams

- Dr. Walter S. Loewe

- Dr. Ralph Mechoulam

You may wonder why knowing who these men are would matter when getting into the habit of using CBD oil. Truth be told, you don't need to know who they are to enjoy using CBD or partake in the various health benefits. The more you know and understand any topic, no matter how small the detail may seem on the surface, can actually go a very long way in bonding you to a product or practice of any kind. Knowing who these people are also showing the reciprocal side of life that you may have let slip by you. Bogging down your busy mind with philosophical rhetoric will not happen here, but it would be good to keep in mind that while you are trying to travel on a voyage and perform an exodus away from the iron like grip of modern medical practices, that the people who discovered and harvested the CBD oil you intend to use were made by scientists.

Odd as it may seem, science is a reflection of nature and there is a give-and-take relationship between man and nature. Remember that scientists and doctors are not the enemies. Technology has no intrinsic nature, no personality, and no moral code. This does not just pertain to our phones, cars, and computers, but all medicine, natural and otherwise as well. It is how the technology is used by men and women that determine something's true value. This pertains to CBD oil and it would be good to remember that CBD oil is also a technology. Yes, it may come from nature but the extraction of it and the various ways that it is used have all the markings of modern technology written all over them.

What are the different methods that CBD oil can be absorbed into the human system?

- CBD oil can be mixed with water or combined with certain foods. Whenever you decide to cook with olive oil, add a little bit of CBD oil to the dish and then enjoy your meal.

- CBD can be taken sublingually, which means that it can be placed under the tongue.

- CBD oil can be taken via tablets that resemble pills. This is an easy method for those first using it or people who want their CBD use to resemble modern day medications.

- CBD oil can be used as a spray that you spritz into the mouth.

- Inhalation. This is the most commonly used method performed via vaping the CBD oil. This is more advanced and may not work best for those just starting out. For others, it is not just the preferred way to receive CBD oil but is also a popular hobby that may even introduce you into an entirely new social circle. There are a large variety of different flavors and devices used for vaping out there, so you may have to take time and do extra research before jumping into the deep ocean of inhaling CBD oil.

- Topical applications can also be used. This is something that everyone should give a go at least once before passing final judgment on it. When CBD oil is used as a cream or lotion, the effects are just immediate. There are many different scents and aromas out there that come along with using CBD oil topical applications. Using CBD oil in this way can also lead you into the world of beauty and skincare if you were interested in looking into that, or already considered yourself a part of it.

- Remember that you can always add CBD oil to a bath. If you decide to only use a trace amount or do the entire bath bomb of CBD oil, either way, you can expect a relaxing soak in the tub.

What are the different types of oils that come from the *Cannabis sativa* plant?

- CBD oil

- Hemp seed oil

- Marijuana oil

- THC oil

- Cannabis oil

What are the different medical conditions that CBD oil can be used to treat?

- Acne

- Epilepsy

- Insomnia

- Anxiety

- Stress

- Depression

- PTSD

- Chron's disease

- Ulcerative colitis

- Glaucoma

- Multiple sclerosis

- Cancer

- Diabetes

- Heart related trouble

- Mania and psychotic behavior

Final Word

Well, that's it. Now you should be more than ready to start using CBD oil. Just remember to work with your health care provider on all medical issues, but no matter what, it will always be up to you to make the final decision for how you want to handle your health.

Conclusion

Thanks for making it through to the end of *CBD OIL: A simple & effective beginner's guide on using CBD Hemp Oil, the natural remedy to cure illnesses, improve health, mental health, pain relief, & cure anxiety without medications*, let's hope it was informative and able to provide you with all of the tools you need to achieve your goals whatever they may be.

The next step is to start learning everything you can about whatever medical affliction you are dealing with. CBD oil can be a powerful weapon to add to your arsenal of health but if you do not know what you are trying to solve, the problem will only continue to linger. As you continue to use CBD oil, and any other holistic remedies, you may not just see yourself growing and feeling healthier but may be inclined to start skipping the visits to the doctor's office. Remember that doctors are not the enemy.

The point of this book has been to give people that are new to the world of CBD oil a starting point that they can build from. Taking your health into your own hands is something you should do but before moving away from the world of modern medicine entirely, make sure that you have a solid foundation of knowledge and understanding regarding CBD oil.

Soon enough you may not need modern medicine anymore. Here's to your health!

Finally, if you found this book useful in any way, a feedback is always appreciated!